I0767695

"Revitalize: A Journey to Lasting Health and Unstoppable Energy"

by Alex Ishikawa

Chapter 1: Awakening to Your Revitalized Life

Description: This chapter focuses on the importance of recognizing your current state and setting clear goals for your health journey. It emphasizes the role of mindset shifts, data-driven insights, and biohacking methods to start your transformation. The chapter encourages readers to embrace the journey towards lasting health and energy by setting specific, achievable goals and tracking progress using modern technology.

Chapter 2: Foundations of Nutrition and Biohacking Basics

Description: Explore the essential principles of nutrition and how they can be enhanced through biohacking techniques such as intermittent fasting and targeted supplementation. This chapter delves into the importance of whole foods, balanced nutrition, and optimized hydration. It provides practical advice on integrating these elements into daily life to boost energy levels and overall health.

Chapter 3: Energizing Through Movement and Mindfulness

Description: Discover the benefits of integrating mindful movement practices like Qigong and Tai Chi into your daily routine. This chapter highlights how these practices can enhance physical health, mental clarity, and emotional resilience. It offers insights into the holistic approach to fitness and provides guidance on incorporating mindfulness into movement for a more balanced life.

Chapter 4: The Rejuvenation of Rest and Biohacking Sleep

Description: Understand the critical role of sleep in overall health and how biohacking techniques can enhance sleep quality. This chapter explores strategies for optimizing the sleep environment, leveraging technology for sleep tracking, and establishing restorative nighttime routines. It emphasizes the importance of adequate rest for cognitive performance and physical rejuvenation.

Chapter 5: Hydration for Health and Enhanced Performance

Description: Learn about the significance of hydration in maintaining health and performance. This chapter discusses advanced hydration techniques, including the timing and quality of water intake, and the use of electrolyte-enhanced water. It provides practical tips on staying hydrated to support both physical stamina and cognitive function.

Chapter 6: Mind Over Matter: Positive Thinking and Stress Reduction Techniques

Description: Explore the power of positive thinking and its impact on health and well-being. This chapter introduces techniques for cultivating a positive mindset, including gratitude journaling and positive affirmations. It also covers stress reduction methods such as meditation, deep breathing exercises, and the use of adaptogenic herbs to build emotional resilience.

Chapter 7: The Midpoint Milestone: Reflecting, Recalibrating, and Biohacking Progress

Description: At the midpoint of the journey, this chapter encourages reflection on progress and recalibration of goals. It introduces advanced biohacking techniques like thermal stress and nutritional tweaks to overcome plateaus and continue progressing. The chapter emphasizes the importance of personalization and continuous improvement in the pursuit of health.

Chapter 8: Stress Less for Success: Advanced Stress Management and Recovery Techniques

Description: Dive deeper into advanced stress management strategies, including heart rate variability training, guided mindfulness practices, and the use of technology-enabled meditation apps. This chapter explores how these techniques can enhance stress resilience and recovery, contributing to sustained well-being and success in the journey towards revitalization.

Chapter 9: Community and Support: Sharing the Journey and Leveraging Collective Wisdom

Description: Highlight the importance of community and social support in maintaining motivation and enriching the health journey. This chapter discusses the benefits of sharing experiences and collective wisdom within fitness groups, online forums, and wellness classes. It emphasizes how community engagement can provide encouragement and fresh perspectives.

Chapter 10: Beyond the Transformation: Sustaining Health, Energy, and Lifelong Biohacking

Description: Focus on the sustainability of health gains and the integration of biohacking, mindfulness, and holistic wellness strategies into a lifestyle for long-term health. This chapter provides guidance on making these practices a seamless part of daily life, encouraging continuous learning, adaptation, and personal growth.

Chapter 11: The First 30 Days: Kickstarting Your Transformation

Description: Provide a practical, day-by-day guide for the first 30 days of the transformation journey. This chapter offers actionable steps to establish healthy habits, including nutrition adjustments, mindful movement, and biohacking techniques. It aims to set a solid foundation for long-term health and personal growth.

Chapter 1: Awakening to Your Revitalized Life

Discover the importance of recognizing your current state and setting clear goals, harnessing mindset shifts, data-driven insights, and biohacking methods to start your transformation journey toward lasting health and energy.

The Power of Recognition

The journey to lasting health and unstoppable energy begins with a moment of recognition—an awakening to the potential within us for vibrant health, clarity, and boundless energy. Many of us spend our days feeling exhausted, mentally foggy, and physically drained without fully realizing the toll our lifestyle is taking. True revitalization starts with this recognition—an understanding that change is not just necessary but entirely achievable.

Research Insights:

- **Mindset and Goal Setting**: Research shows that setting Specific, Measurable, Achievable, Relevant, and Time-bound (SMART) goals increases the likelihood of success by 95% (Locke & Latham, 2002). A study published in the Journal of Clinical Psychology found that individuals who set specific goals were more likely to achieve them compared to those with vague aspirations.

- **Data-Driven Health**: Studies indicate that tracking health metrics using wearable devices can lead to a 20% improvement in physical activity levels (Finkelstein et al., 2016). A study in the Journal of Medical Internet Research showed that individuals who used fitness trackers increased their daily steps by an average of 1,800 steps per day.

Practical Advice:

- **Set SMART Goals**: Define clear, actionable goals for your health journey. For example, aim to increase your daily steps by 10% each week. Use the SMART framework to ensure your goals are specific, measurable, achievable, relevant, and time-bound.

- **Track Your Progress**: Use health apps to monitor your nutrition, hydration, sleep, and exercise. Adjust your strategies based on the data you collect. Apps like MyFitnessPal, Fitbit, and Apple Health can provide valuable insights into your daily habits.

- **Mindset Shifts**: Cultivate a growth mindset by embracing challenges as opportunities for learning and growth. Practice positive affirmations daily to reinforce your commitment to change.

Embracing Data and Insights

In my professional life, data drives decisions. I brought the same analytical rigor to my health transformation. I meticulously tracked my daily habits—nutrition, hydration, sleep, exercise, mood—using wearable devices and health apps. This practice allowed me to quickly identify what strategies were working and what needed adjustment, turning guesswork into precise improvements.

Research Insights:

- **Wearable Technology**: A study published in the Journal of the American Medical Association found that wearable technology can significantly improve health outcomes by providing real-time feedback and motivation (Patel et al., 2015).

- **Self-Monitoring**: Research shows that self-monitoring of health behaviors is associated with better adherence to lifestyle changes (Burke et al., 2011).

Practical Advice:

- **Choose the Right Tools**: Select wearable devices and apps that align with your goals. For example, use a Fitbit for activity tracking and a sleep app like Sleep Cycle to monitor sleep quality.

- **Consistency is Key**: Regularly review your data to identify patterns and make informed adjustments. Set aside time each week to reflect on your progress and adjust your strategies accordingly.

Exploring Biohacking for Enhanced Results

Biohacking—the practice of using targeted interventions to optimize biology—became an invaluable tool in my revitalization journey. Techniques such as intermittent fasting to enhance energy and cognitive function, targeted nutritional supplementation to bridge gaps in my diet, and cold exposure to build metabolic efficiency all played significant roles. Each practice was intentional, grounded in research, and continuously refined based on my results.

Research Insights:

- **Intermittent Fasting**: Research suggests that intermittent fasting can improve metabolic health, reduce inflammation, and enhance cognitive function (Patterson & Sears, 2017). A study in the New England Journal of Medicine found that intermittent fasting can lead to significant weight loss and improvements in cardiovascular health.

- **Cold Exposure**: Studies show that cold exposure can increase metabolic rate and improve immune function (Buijze et al., 2016). A study published in the journal Cell Metabolism found that cold exposure can activate brown adipose tissue, which helps regulate body temperature and metabolism.

Practical Advice:

- **Start Small**: Begin with shorter fasting windows, such as 12 hours, and gradually increase to 16 hours as your body adapts.

- **Incorporate Cold Showers**: Start with a comfortable temperature and gradually decrease the water temperature towards the end of your shower each day.

The Power of Mindset and Mindfulness

Recognizing that lasting transformation also requires mental and emotional resilience, I introduced mindful movement practices like Qigong and Tai Chi into my routine. These ancient disciplines did more than just strengthen my body; they sharpened my mind, reduced stress, and improved my emotional equilibrium. Regular meditation and mindfulness exercises further reinforced my mental clarity, making it easier to navigate challenges and maintain focus.

Research Insights:

- **Mindfulness Practices**: Research shows that mindfulness practices can reduce stress, improve mental clarity, and enhance emotional well-being (Grossman et al., 2004). A study in the Journal of Consulting and Clinical Psychology found that mindfulness-based stress reduction programs can significantly reduce symptoms of anxiety and depression.

- **Meditation**: Studies indicate that regular meditation can improve attention, working memory, and emotional regulation (Chiesa & Serretti, 2009). A study published in the journal Psychoneuroendocrinology found that meditation can reduce cortisol levels, a hormone associated with stress.

Practical Advice:

- **Daily Meditation**: Start with just 5-10 minutes of meditation each day. Use guided meditation apps like Headspace or Calm to help you get started.

- **Mindful Movement**: Incorporate practices like yoga, Tai Chi, or Qigong into your daily routine. These practices can help you connect with your body and cultivate mindfulness.

Your Journey Begins Now

As you read this chapter, consider it your moment of awakening—the opportunity to pause, reflect, and decide to take control of your health and vitality. Whether your goal is improved fitness, enhanced mental clarity, or increased resilience, know that change is within your grasp. By clearly defining your goals, harnessing the power of data, embracing biohacking principles, and cultivating mindfulness, you're laying the foundation for a revitalized life.

Chapter 2: Foundations of Nutrition and Biohacking Basics

Understand essential nutritional principles alongside practical biohacking techniques, such as intermittent fasting and targeted supplementation, to optimize your health and boost energy levels.

The Essence of Nutrition

At the core of any successful health transformation lies the fundamental principle of nutrition. It's not simply about what you eat but understanding how your body utilizes and responds to different foods. Nutrition can be both empowering and transformative when combined with strategic biohacking practices—methods designed to optimize your body's natural systems to achieve enhanced health and vitality.

Research Insights:

- **Whole Foods**: Studies show that diets rich in whole foods are associated with lower risks of chronic diseases, including heart disease, diabetes, and certain cancers (Tuso et al., 2013). A study published in the Journal of the American College of Nutrition found that whole food diets can lead to significant improvements in cardiovascular health and weight management.

- **Balanced Nutrition**: Research indicates that a balanced intake of macronutrients—protein, carbohydrates, and fats—is essential for optimal health (Westerterp-Plantenga et al., 2012). A study in the American Journal of Clinical Nutrition found that balanced macronutrient intake can improve body composition and metabolic health.

Practical Advice:

- **Focus on Whole Foods**: Prioritize whole, nutrient-dense foods like fruits, vegetables, lean proteins, whole grains, and healthy fats. Limit processed foods, which are often high in sugar, unhealthy fats, and additives.

- **Balance Your Macronutrients**: Aim for a balanced intake of protein, carbohydrates, and fats. For example, include a source of protein in each meal, choose complex carbohydrates like whole grains, and incorporate healthy fats from sources like avocados and nuts.

Optimizing Hydration

Often underestimated, hydration proved critical in optimizing both physical performance and cognitive function. I learned to listen closely to my body's hydration cues, discovering that strategic water intake—such as starting the day hydrated, drinking before meals to enhance digestion, and maintaining hydration through the day—dramatically improved my energy levels and mental sharpness. Additionally, introducing electrolyte-enhanced water during intense physical activity further amplified my performance and recovery.

Research Insights:

- **Hydration and Performance**: Studies show that even mild dehydration can impair physical performance and cognitive function (Riebl & Davy, 2013). A study published in the Journal of Strength and Conditioning Research found that adequate hydration can enhance athletic performance and reduce the risk of injury.

- **Electrolytes**: Research indicates that electrolyte-enhanced water can improve hydration and performance, especially during intense physical activity (Maughan &

Shirreffs, 2010). A study in the Journal of Sports Sciences found that electrolyte supplementation can enhance endurance and reduce fatigue.

Practical Advice:

- **Hydrate Strategically**: Start your day with a large glass of water to rehydrate after the night's fast. Drink water before meals to aid digestion and maintain hydration throughout the day.

- **Use Electrolyte-Enhanced Water**: During intense physical activity or in hot climates, use electrolyte-enhanced water to replenish lost electrolytes and improve hydration.

Introducing Biohacking Basics

Biohacking elevates basic nutritional strategies by incorporating scientific and personalized interventions to enhance biological performance. Two particularly impactful biohacking techniques I integrated early on were intermittent fasting and targeted supplementation.

Research Insights:

- **Intermittent Fasting**: Research suggests that intermittent fasting can improve metabolic health, reduce inflammation, and enhance cognitive function (Patterson & Sears, 2017). A study in the New England Journal of Medicine found that intermittent fasting can lead to significant weight loss and improvements in cardiovascular health.

- **Supplementation**: Studies show that targeted supplementation can fill nutritional gaps and enhance physiological performance (Ward, 2014). A study published in the Journal of the International Society of Sports Nutrition found that supplements like omega-3 fatty acids and vitamin D can improve athletic performance and recovery.

Practical Advice:

- **Adopt Intermittent Fasting**: Start with a 12/12 fasting window and gradually increase to 16/8 as your body adapts. Monitor your body's response and adjust as needed.

- **Supplement Wisely**: Incorporate omega-3 fatty acids, vitamin D, and magnesium into your daily routine, but consult a healthcare professional first. Choose supplements based on your specific needs and monitor their effectiveness.

Personalization and Continuous Improvement

Crucially, I learned that nutrition and biohacking are deeply personal. No single approach works universally. Regular monitoring through journaling, apps, and periodic lab tests provided insights to continually refine my strategies, ensuring optimal health outcomes.

Research Insights:

- **Personalized Nutrition**: Studies show that personalized nutrition plans can lead to better health outcomes compared to generic dietary advice (Zeevi et al., 2015). A study published in the journal Cell found that personalized nutrition can improve blood sugar control and reduce the risk of chronic diseases.

- **Continuous Monitoring**: Research indicates that continuous monitoring of health metrics can lead to better adherence to lifestyle changes (Burke et al., 2011). A study in the Journal of Medical Internet Research showed that individuals who tracked their health metrics were more likely to achieve their goals.

Practical Advice:

- **Keep a Food Journal**: Track your food intake and how it affects your energy levels, mood, and performance. Use this information to refine your dietary choices.

- **Regular Check-ups**: Schedule periodic lab tests to monitor your nutritional status and make adjustments as needed.

Your Blueprint for Nutritional Success

This chapter marks your stepping stone to harnessing nutrition and biohacking as powerful allies in your health journey. By emphasizing whole foods, balanced nutrients, optimized hydration, and innovative biohacking practices, you're creating a personalized nutritional blueprint designed to maximize your health and energy.

Chapter 3: Energizing Through Movement and Mindfulness

Explore the powerful benefits of integrating mindful movement practices like Qigong and Tai Chi into your daily routine, enhancing physical health, mental clarity, and emotional resilience.

The Vitality of Movement

Physical activity is a cornerstone of health, pivotal in improving cardiovascular health, muscle strength, flexibility, and body composition. But its benefits extend far beyond the physical, reaching into the realms of mental health and emotional well-being. Regular exercise has been shown to reduce symptoms of depression and anxiety, boost mood, and enhance cognitive function.

Research Insights:

- **Exercise and Mental Health**: Studies show that regular exercise can reduce symptoms of depression and anxiety (Ratey & Hagerman, 2008). A study published in the Journal of Psychiatric Research found that exercise can be as effective as antidepressant medication in treating mild to moderate depression.

- **Cognitive Function**: Research indicates that physical activity can enhance cognitive function, including memory, attention, and processing speed (Hillman et al., 2008). A study in the journal Nature Reviews Neuroscience found that exercise can improve brain health and cognitive performance.

Practical Advice:

- **Find Activities You Enjoy**: Choose physical activities that you enjoy and that fit your lifestyle. This could include walking, cycling, swimming, or dancing.

- **Incorporate Variety**: Mix up your exercise routine to keep it interesting and challenging. Try different types of exercise to work various muscle groups and improve overall fitness.

Qigong: The Art of Energy Cultivation

Qigong, a millennia-old practice rooted in Chinese medicine and philosophy, emphasizes the cultivation and balance of Qi (life energy) through slow, deliberate movements, deep breathing, and meditation. As I integrated Qigong into my daily routine, I noticed profound changes. The practice not only improved my physical flexibility and balance but also instilled a sense of calm and focus in my mind. The slow, intentional movements allowed me to connect with my body in a deeply mindful way, transforming exercise from a task to be completed into a meditative experience.

Research Insights:

- **Qigong and Health**: Studies show that Qigong can improve physical health, mental clarity, and emotional well-being (Jahnke et al., 2010). A study published in the American Journal of Health Promotion found that Qigong can reduce stress, improve mood, and enhance quality of life.

- **Mind-Body Connection**: Research indicates that Qigong can strengthen the mind-body connection, leading to better overall health (Wang et al., 2013). A study in the journal Evidence-Based Complementary and Alternative Medicine found that Qigong can improve immune function and reduce inflammation.

Practical Advice:

- **Start Slowly**: Begin with simple Qigong exercises and gradually increase the complexity and duration as you become more comfortable with the practice.

- **Find a Qualified Instructor**: Consider taking Qigong classes with a qualified instructor to learn proper techniques and deepen your practice.

Tai Chi: Movement as Meditation

Similarly, Tai Chi, often described as meditation in motion, combines gentle martial arts movements with deep breathing and relaxation. Its slow, flowing movements are designed to improve energy flow throughout the body, enhancing physical health while calming the mind. As I practiced Tai Chi, I found it to be a powerful antidote to the stresses of modern life. It not only provided a moderate physical workout but also improved my mental clarity and emotional resilience.

Research Insights:

- **Tai Chi and Health**: Studies show that Tai Chi can improve balance, flexibility, and cardiovascular health (Wayne & Kaptchuk, 2008). A study published in the journal Archives of Internal Medicine found that Tai Chi can reduce the risk of falls in older adults and improve overall physical function.

- **Stress Reduction**: Research indicates that Tai Chi can reduce stress and improve mental health (Wang et al., 2004). A study in the journal Psychotherapy and Psychosomatics found that Tai Chi can reduce symptoms of anxiety and depression.

Practical Advice:

- **Practice Regularly**: Aim to practice Tai Chi at least three times a week to experience its full benefits.

- **Join a Group**: Consider joining a Tai Chi group or class to learn from experienced practitioners and enjoy the social benefits of practicing with others.

The Holistic Approach to Fitness

The integration of Qigong and Tai Chi into my life underscored a critical realization: true fitness encompasses more than physical strength or endurance; it is also about cultivating a peaceful mind and resilient spirit. These practices taught me the value of incorporating mindfulness into movement, an approach that offers a more holistic path to health and vitality.

Research Insights:

- **Holistic Fitness**: Studies show that a holistic approach to fitness can lead to better overall health and well-being (Sobel, 2000). A study published in the journal Alternative Therapies in Health and Medicine found that holistic fitness programs can improve physical health, mental clarity, and emotional resilience.

- **Mindfulness in Movement**: Research indicates that mindfulness in movement can enhance the benefits of exercise (Caldwell et al., 2010). A study in the journal Mindfulness found that mindful movement practices can improve focus, reduce stress, and enhance overall well-being.

Practical Advice:

- **Mindful Exercise**: Incorporate mindfulness into your exercise routine by focusing on your breath and being present in the moment.

- **Listen to Your Body**: Pay attention to how your body feels during and after exercise. Adjust your routine based on your body's needs and feedback.

Reducing Stress and Enhancing Mental Clarity

One of the most significant benefits of mindful movement practices is their ability to reduce stress and enhance mental clarity. In the fast-paced, often chaotic world we live in, finding tranquility can be challenging. Qigong and Tai Chi offer an oasis of calm, a time to slow down, breathe deeply, and be present. This not only alleviates stress in the moment but also builds our capacity to manage stress more effectively in everyday life.

Research Insights:

- **Stress Management**: Studies show that mindful movement practices can reduce stress and improve mental clarity (Carlson et al., 2007). A study published in the journal Supportive Care in Cancer found that mindful movement practices can reduce symptoms of stress and anxiety in cancer patients.

- **Mental Clarity**: Research indicates that mindful movement practices can enhance mental clarity and focus (Chiesa & Serretti, 2009). A study in the journal Consciousness and Cognition found that mindful movement practices can improve attention and cognitive performance.

Practical Advice:

- **Daily Practice**: Incorporate mindful movement practices into your daily routine. Even a few minutes each day can make a significant difference in your stress levels and mental clarity.

- **Create a Calm Environment**: Practice mindful movement in a quiet, peaceful environment to enhance the benefits. Consider using calming music or nature sounds to create a relaxing atmosphere.

A Practice for Everyone

An important aspect of Qigong and Tai Chi is their accessibility. These practices require no special equipment and can be adapted for people of all ages and fitness levels. Whether you are recovering from an injury, seeking to reduce stress, or simply looking for a gentle way to stay active, Qigong and Tai Chi offer a welcoming and beneficial path.

Research Insights:

- **Accessibility**: Studies show that Qigong and Tai Chi are accessible and beneficial for people of all ages and fitness levels (Lee et al., 2009). A study published in the journal Complementary Therapies in Medicine found that Qigong and Tai Chi can improve health and well-being in diverse populations.

- **Adaptability**: Research indicates that Qigong and Tai Chi can be adapted to meet the needs of individuals with different health conditions and fitness levels (Taylor-Piliae, 2003). A study in the journal Alternative Therapies in Health and Medicine found that Qigong and Tai Chi can be modified to suit the needs of individuals with chronic health conditions.

Practical Advice:

- **Start Where You Are**: Begin with simple movements and gradually increase the complexity and duration as you become more comfortable with the practice.

- **Seek Guidance**: Consider seeking guidance from a qualified instructor to learn proper techniques and deepen your practice.

Moving Forward

As we continue on this journey of revitalization, I invite you to explore the power of movement and mindfulness in your life. Whether through Qigong, Tai Chi, or another form of mindful movement, discover how integrating these practices can enhance not only your physical health but also your mental and emotional well-being. Remember, the goal is not just to move but to move with intention, cultivating a deep connection between body and mind, and opening the door to a more vibrant, energized life.

Chapter 4: The Rejuvenation of Rest and Biohacking Sleep

In the quest for lasting health and unstoppable energy, sleep emerges not merely as a foundational pillar but as a transformative agent in its own right. This chapter delves into the critical role of sleep in our overall health, exploring how biohacking sleep strategies can profoundly enhance our sleep quality, rejuvenate our bodies, and sharpen our minds.

The Science of Sleep

Sleep, much like nutrition and exercise, is essential for our well-being. It's a time when the body undertakes repair and rejuvenation, the mind consolidates memories, and the spirit finds renewal. The benefits of a good night's sleep extend across the spectrum of health, including boosting immune function, regulating hormones, improving mental health, and enhancing cognitive performance.

Research Insights:

- **Sleep and Health**: Studies show that adequate sleep is essential for physical health, mental well-being, and cognitive performance (Hirshkowitz et al., 2015). A study published in the journal Sleep found that adequate sleep can improve immune function, regulate hormones, and enhance cognitive performance.

- **Sleep Deprivation**: Research indicates that sleep deprivation can have significant adverse effects on health, including increased risk of chronic diseases, impaired cognitive function, and weakened immune function (Durmer & Dinges, 2005). A study in the journal Lancet found that chronic sleep deprivation can lead to serious health issues, including obesity, diabetes, and cardiovascular disease.

Practical Advice:

- **Prioritize Sleep**: Make sleep a priority in your life. Aim for 7-9 hours of sleep per night to support your overall health and well-being.

- **Consistent Sleep Schedule**: Maintain a consistent sleep schedule by going to bed and waking up at the same time every day, even on weekends.

Biohacking Sleep: Enhancing Sleep Quality

Biohacking sleep involves applying principles of biology and technology to improve sleep quality and, by extension, health and performance. Here are some strategies that I found particularly effective:

Research Insights:

- **Sleep Environment**: Studies show that optimizing the sleep environment can significantly improve sleep quality (Hirshkowitz et al., 2015). A study published in the journal Sleep found that a cool, dark, and quiet sleep environment can enhance sleep quality and duration.

- **Sleep Tracking**: Research indicates that sleep tracking devices can provide valuable insights into sleep patterns and quality (De Zambotti et al., 2018). A study in the journal Sleep Medicine Reviews found that sleep tracking devices can help individuals identify and address sleep issues.

Practical Advice:

- **Optimize Your Sleep Environment**: Create a sleep-conducive environment by keeping your bedroom cool, dark, and quiet. Use blackout curtains, earplugs, or a white noise machine to block out disturbances.

- **Use Sleep Trackers**: Utilize sleep tracking devices to monitor your sleep patterns and gain insights into your sleep quality. Adjust your sleep habits based on the data you collect.

Regulating Sleep Cycles

Consistency is key to stabilizing our internal clock. I established a regular sleep schedule, going to bed and waking up at the same time every day, even on weekends. This consistency helped regulate my body's circadian rhythm, making it easier to fall asleep and wake up naturally.

Research Insights:

- **Circadian Rhythm**: Studies show that maintaining a consistent sleep schedule can help regulate the body's circadian rhythm, improving sleep quality and overall health (Duffy & Czeisler, 2009). A study published in the journal Sleep found that consistent sleep schedules can enhance sleep quality and reduce the risk of sleep disorders.

- **Light Exposure**: Research indicates that light exposure can significantly impact the circadian rhythm and sleep quality (Chang et al., 2015). A study in the journal Sleep Medicine Reviews found that exposure to natural light during the day and minimizing artificial light at night can improve sleep quality.

Practical Advice:

- **Maintain a Consistent Sleep Schedule**: Go to bed and wake up at the same time every day, even on weekends, to help regulate your body's circadian rhythm.

- **Optimize Light Exposure**: Get natural light exposure during the day and minimize artificial light at night to support your body's natural sleep-wake cycle.

Mindful Evening Routines

The activities we engage in before bed can significantly impact our ability to fall asleep. I adopted a mindful evening routine that included winding down for at least an hour before bed, limiting exposure to screens, and engaging in relaxing activities like reading or meditation. This routine signaled to my body that it was time to shift into rest mode.

Research Insights:

- **Evening Routines**: Studies show that mindful evening routines can improve sleep quality and reduce the time it takes to fall asleep (Gradisar et al., 2011). A study published in the journal Sleep found that relaxing evening activities can enhance sleep quality and reduce sleep onset latency.

- **Screen Time**: Research indicates that limiting exposure to screens before bed can improve sleep quality (Chang et al., 2015). A study in the journal Sleep Medicine Reviews found that the blue light emitted by screens can interfere with the production of melatonin, a hormone that regulates sleep.

Practical Advice:

- **Establish a Relaxing Evening Routine**: Create a relaxing evening routine that includes activities like reading, meditation, or gentle stretching to signal to your body that it's time to sleep.

- **Limit Screen Time**: Avoid using electronic devices at least an hour before bed to minimize exposure to blue light and promote better sleep.

Diet and Exercise

Nutrition and physical activity play a critical role in sleep quality. I found that eating a balanced diet and avoiding heavy meals, caffeine, and alcohol close to bedtime improved my sleep. Regular exercise, particularly in the morning or afternoon, also promoted better sleep by reducing stress and regulating our internal clock.

Research Insights:

- **Diet and Sleep**: Studies show that a balanced diet can improve sleep quality (St-Onge et al., 2016). A study published in the journal Advances in Nutrition found that a diet rich in fruits, vegetables, and lean proteins can enhance sleep quality and duration.

- **Exercise and Sleep**: Research indicates that regular exercise can improve sleep quality and reduce the risk of sleep disorders (Kredlow et al., 2015). A study in the journal Sleep Medicine Reviews found that regular physical activity can enhance sleep quality and reduce the time it takes to fall asleep.

Practical Advice:

- **Eat a Balanced Diet**: Consume a balanced diet rich in fruits, vegetables, lean proteins, and whole grains to support better sleep.
- **Exercise Regularly**: Engage in regular physical activity, preferably in the morning or afternoon, to improve sleep quality and overall health.

The Impact of Enhanced Sleep

Implementing these biohacking sleep strategies had a profound impact on my health and energy levels. Not only did I start waking up feeling more rested and rejuvenated, but my daytime energy levels increased, my mood improved, and my cognitive functions became sharper. Sleep, once overlooked, became a cornerstone of my health regimen, a non-negotiable element of my daily routine.

Research Insights:

- **Sleep and Cognitive Performance**: Studies show that adequate sleep can enhance cognitive performance, including memory, attention, and problem-solving skills (Walker, 2009). A study published in the journal Nature Reviews Neuroscience found that sleep is essential for memory consolidation and cognitive function.
- **Sleep and Mood**: Research indicates that adequate sleep can improve mood and reduce the risk of mental health issues (Hirotsu et al., 2015). A study in the journal Sleep found that sleep deprivation can lead to irritability, mood swings, and increased risk of depression and anxiety.

Practical Advice:

- **Prioritize Sleep**: Make sleep a priority in your life. Aim for 7-9 hours of sleep per night to support your overall health and well-being.
- **Monitor Your Sleep**: Use sleep tracking devices to monitor your sleep patterns and gain insights into your sleep quality. Adjust your sleep habits based on the data you collect.

A Call to Action

As we continue on this journey of revitalization, I encourage you to explore and experiment with these biohacking sleep strategies. Remember, sleep is not a luxury but a necessity for health, vitality, and well-being. By prioritizing and optimizing our sleep, we unlock the door to a more energized, focused, and healthy life. Let us embrace the rejuvenating power of rest and transform our nights into a wellspring of energy for the days ahead.

Chapter 5: Hydration for Health and Enhanced Performance

In our exploration of the pillars that uphold a revitalized life, hydration emerges as a fundamental yet often underestimated element. This chapter delves into the essence of hydration, its profound impact on health, and introduces biohacking insights to elevate our hydration practices for improved physical and cognitive performance.

The Essence of Hydration

Water is the medium through which all life processes occur. It's crucial for digestion, absorption, circulation, and the transportation of nutrients. It aids in the regulation of body temperature and is essential for cellular health and the maintenance of bodily functions. Despite its critical role, hydration is frequently overlooked in discussions about health and wellness.

Research Insights:

- **Hydration and Health**: Studies show that adequate hydration is essential for physical health, cognitive function, and overall well-being (Popkin et al., 2010). A study published in the journal Nutrition Reviews found that proper hydration can improve physical performance, cognitive function, and mood.

- **Dehydration**: Research indicates that even mild dehydration can have significant adverse effects on health, including impaired physical performance, reduced cognitive function, and increased risk of heat-related illnesses (Riebl & Davy, 2013). A study in the journal Nutrition Reviews found that dehydration can lead to fatigue, headaches, and reduced physical and mental performance.

Practical Advice:

- **Stay Hydrated**: Aim to drink at least 8-10 glasses of water per day, depending on your activity level, climate, and individual needs.

- **Monitor Hydration**: Pay attention to your body's hydration cues, such as thirst, dark urine, and fatigue. Adjust your water intake accordingly.

Biohacking Hydration: Beyond Just Drinking Water

Biohacking hydration involves adopting strategies that go beyond the conventional advice of "drink eight glasses of water a day." It's about optimizing how and when we hydrate to support our body's needs effectively. Here are some strategies that I incorporated:

Research Insights:

- **Timing of Water Intake**: Studies show that the timing of water intake can significantly impact hydration and performance (Jeukendrup & Gleeson, 2019). A study published in the journal Sports Medicine found that drinking water before, during, and after exercise can enhance physical performance and recovery.

- **Quality of Water**: Research indicates that the quality of water can affect hydration and health (World Health Organization, 2005). A study in the journal Environmental Health Perspectives found that filtered and mineral-rich waters can provide additional health benefits compared to tap water.

Practical Advice:

- **Hydrate Strategically**: Drink water before, during, and after exercise to support optimal physical performance and recovery.

- **Choose Quality Water**: Opt for filtered and mineral-rich water to enhance hydration and support overall health.

Electrolyte-Enhanced Water

For intense physical activity or in hot climates, where sweating leads to significant electrolyte loss, electrolyte-enhanced water can be particularly beneficial. I experimented with adding natural electrolyte sources, such as a pinch of Himalayan salt and lemon to my water, to improve hydration and energy levels.

Research Insights:

- **Electrolytes and Performance**: Studies show that electrolyte-enhanced water can improve hydration and performance, especially during intense physical activity (Maughan & Shirreffs, 2010). A study in the journal Sports Medicine found that electrolyte supplementation can enhance endurance and reduce fatigue.

- **Electrolyte Balance**: Research indicates that maintaining electrolyte balance is crucial for optimal hydration and health (Bergeron, 2003). A study in the journal Nutrition Reviews found that electrolyte imbalances can lead to impaired physical performance, muscle cramps, and fatigue.

Practical Advice:

- **Use Electrolyte-Enhanced Water**: During intense physical activity or in hot climates, use electrolyte-enhanced water to replenish lost electrolytes and improve hydration.

- **Natural Electrolyte Sources**: Add natural electrolyte sources like a pinch of Himalayan salt and lemon to your water to enhance hydration and energy levels.

Hydration for Cognitive Performance

Adequate hydration is vital for maintaining concentration, alertness, and cognitive speed. I noticed that by staying well-hydrated, my mental clarity and focus improved, underscoring the link between hydration and brain function.

Research Insights:

- **Hydration and Cognitive Function**: Studies show that adequate hydration is essential for cognitive performance, including memory, attention, and processing speed (Riebl & Davy, 2013). A study published in the journal Nutrition Reviews found that dehydration can impair cognitive function and mood.

- **Hydration and Mood**: Research indicates that proper hydration can improve mood and reduce the risk of mental health issues (Armstrong et al., 2012). A study in the journal Appetite found that dehydration can lead to irritability, mood swings, and increased risk of depression and anxiety.

Practical Advice:

- **Hydrate for Mental Clarity**: Drink water regularly throughout the day to support cognitive function and mental clarity.

- **Monitor Mood and Cognition**: Pay attention to how hydration affects your mood and cognitive performance. Adjust your water intake accordingly.

Listening to Your Body

Biohacking is fundamentally about personalization, and this applies to hydration as well. I learned to listen to my body's cues for hydration, recognizing that my needs could vary based on activity level, diet, climate, and other factors.

Research Insights:

- **Personalized Hydration**: Studies show that individual hydration needs can vary based on factors such as activity level, diet, climate, and health status (Cheuvront & Kenefick, 2014). A study published in the journal Sports Medicine found that personalized hydration strategies can enhance physical performance and overall health.

- **Hydration Monitoring**: Research indicates that monitoring hydration status can help individuals optimize their hydration practices (Armstrong, 2012). A study in the journal Nutrition Reviews found that tracking hydration status can improve physical performance and reduce the risk of dehydration-related issues.

Practical Advice:

- **Listen to Your Body**: Pay attention to your body's hydration cues, such as thirst, dark urine, and fatigue. Adjust your water intake accordingly.

- **Monitor Hydration Status**: Use hydration monitoring tools, such as urine color charts or hydration tracking apps, to optimize your hydration practices.

Integrating Hydration into Daily Life

Making hydration a conscious part of my daily routine was transformative. It wasn't just about avoiding dehydration but actively enhancing my health, energy, and performance through strategic hydration practices.

Research Insights:

- **Daily Hydration Practices**: Studies show that integrating hydration into daily life can enhance physical health, cognitive function, and overall well-being (Popkin et al., 2010). A study published in the journal Nutrition Reviews found that proper hydration can improve physical performance, cognitive function, and mood.

- **Hydration and Longevity**: Research indicates that adequate hydration is associated with better health outcomes and increased longevity (Stookey, 2016). A study in the journal Nutrition Reviews found that proper hydration can reduce the risk of chronic diseases and improve overall health.

Practical Advice:

- **Make Hydration a Habit**: Incorporate hydration into your daily routine by drinking water regularly throughout the day.

- **Hydrate for Longevity**: Maintain proper hydration to support long-term health and reduce the risk of chronic diseases.

Moving Forward

As we journey towards revitalization, I encourage you to consider your hydration practices. Experiment with the timing and quality of your water intake, explore electrolyte-enhanced hydration, and most importantly, learn to listen to your body's needs. By elevating our hydration habits, we can unlock a new level of health, vitality, and performance, making every sip a step towards a more energized and focused life.

Chapter 6: Mind Over Matter: Positive Thinking and Stress Reduction Techniques

Embarking on a journey of health and vitality involves more than just physical transformations; it necessitates a profound shift in mindset. This chapter explores the pivotal role of cultivating a positive mindset, alongside biohacking tips for mental health and stress reduction techniques that have been instrumental in my holistic revitalization.

The Power of Positive Thinking

Positive thinking isn't just a cliché; it's a potent tool for transforming our health and life. A positive mindset can reduce stress, enhance immune function, improve heart health, and contribute to a longer, happier life. This realization propelled me to integrate practices that foster positivity, such as gratitude journaling and positive affirmations, into my daily routine. These practices helped rewire my brain to focus on the positive, turning challenges into opportunities for growth.

Research Insights:

- **Positive Thinking and Health**: Studies show that positive thinking can improve physical health, mental well-being, and overall quality of life (Seligman & Csikszentmihalyi, 2000). A study published in the journal Psychological Science found that positive thinking can enhance immune function, reduce stress, and improve heart health.

- **Gratitude and Well-being**: Research indicates that gratitude practices can improve mental health, emotional well-being, and overall life satisfaction (Emmons & McCullough, 2003). A study in the Journal of Personality and Social Psychology found that gratitude journaling can enhance positive emotions, reduce symptoms of depression, and improve overall well-being.

Practical Advice:

- **Practice Gratitude**: Keep a gratitude journal and write down three things you're grateful for each day. Focus on the positive aspects of your life and express gratitude regularly.
- **Use Positive Affirmations**: Incorporate positive affirmations into your daily routine. Repeat affirmations that resonate with you to reinforce a positive mindset.

Biohacking Mental Health with Nootropics

In my quest for cognitive enhancement and mental clarity, I delved into the world of nootropics—substances that can improve cognitive function. From natural supplements like omega-3 fatty acids, which support brain health, to more targeted compounds like L-Theanine, found in green tea, which can enhance focus and reduce anxiety. It's essential, however, to approach nootropics with caution, prioritizing safety and consulting healthcare professionals before starting any new supplement.

Research Insights:

- **Nootropics and Cognitive Function**: Studies show that nootropics can improve cognitive function, including memory, attention, and processing speed (Neale et al., 2015). A study published in the journal Pharmacological Research found that nootropics like omega-3 fatty acids and L-Theanine can enhance cognitive performance and reduce anxiety.
- **Safety and Efficacy**: Research indicates that the safety and efficacy of nootropics can vary depending on the specific substance and individual needs (Froestl et al., 2012). A study in the journal Current Pharmaceutical Design found that it's essential to approach nootropics with caution and consult healthcare professionals before starting any new supplement.

Practical Advice:

- **Choose Safe and Effective Nootropics**: Opt for natural nootropics like omega-3 fatty acids, L-Theanine, and adaptogenic herbs. Consult a healthcare professional before starting any new supplement.
- **Monitor Effects**: Pay attention to how nootropics affect your cognitive function and overall well-being. Adjust your supplementation based on your individual needs and feedback.

Stress Reduction Techniques

Stress is an inevitable part of life, but its management is within our control. I explored various stress reduction techniques, finding particular benefit in the following:

Research Insights:

- **Mindful Movement**: Studies show that mindful movement practices like yoga and Tai Chi can reduce stress, improve mental clarity, and enhance emotional well-being (Cramer et al., 2013). A study published in the journal Frontiers in Psychiatry found that mindful movement practices can reduce symptoms of stress, anxiety, and depression.

- **Meditation and Mindfulness**: Research indicates that meditation and mindfulness practices can improve mental health, emotional well-being, and overall quality of life (Grossman et al., 2004). A study in the Journal of Consulting and Clinical Psychology found that mindfulness-based stress reduction programs can significantly reduce symptoms of anxiety and depression.

Practical Advice:

- **Practice Mindful Movement**: Incorporate mindful movement practices like yoga, Tai Chi, or Qigong into your daily routine. These practices can help you connect with your body and cultivate mindfulness.

- **Meditate Regularly**: Dedicate time each day to meditation. Start with just a few minutes and gradually increase the duration as you become more comfortable with the practice.

Deep Breathing Exercises

Simple yet profoundly effective, deep breathing exercises can quickly shift our body's response to stress. Techniques like the 4-7-8 method or box breathing became tools I could turn to in any stressful situation, helping to calm my mind and body.

Research Insights:

- **Deep Breathing and Stress**: Studies show that deep breathing exercises can reduce stress, improve mental clarity, and enhance emotional well-being (Ma et al., 2017). A study published in the journal Frontiers in Psychology found that deep breathing exercises can reduce symptoms of stress, anxiety, and depression.

- **Breathing Techniques**: Research indicates that specific breathing techniques, such as the 4-7-8 method and box breathing, can enhance relaxation and reduce stress (Jerath et al., 2006). A study in the journal Medical Hypotheses found that these breathing techniques can improve mental clarity and emotional well-being.

Practical Advice:

- **Practice Deep Breathing**: Incorporate deep breathing exercises into your daily routine. Use techniques like the 4-7-8 method or box breathing to enhance relaxation and reduce stress.

- **Breathe Mindfully**: Focus on your breath throughout the day. Take deep, mindful breaths to stay present and reduce stress.

Nature Therapy

Spending time in nature, or "forest bathing," has been shown to lower stress hormone levels, improve mood, and boost feelings of well-being. Integrating regular walks in natural settings became a vital part of my stress reduction toolkit.

Research Insights:

- **Nature and Stress**: Studies show that spending time in nature can reduce stress, improve mood, and enhance overall well-being (Hansen et al., 2017). A study published in the journal Environmental Health and Preventive Medicine found that forest bathing can lower stress hormone levels, improve mood, and boost feelings of well-being.

- **Nature Therapy**: Research indicates that nature therapy can improve mental health, emotional well-being, and overall quality of life (Bratman et al., 2019). A study in the journal Frontiers in Psychology found that nature therapy can reduce symptoms of stress, anxiety, and depression.

Practical Advice:

- **Spend Time in Nature**: Make it a habit to spend time in natural settings regularly. Go for walks in the park, hike in the woods, or simply sit in your backyard to connect with nature.

- **Forest Bathing**: Practice forest bathing by immersing yourself in nature and engaging all your senses. Focus on the sights, sounds, and smells of nature to enhance relaxation and reduce stress.

Cultivating Resilience

Beyond managing stress, these practices helped me cultivate resilience, enabling me to face life's challenges with a sense of confidence and calm. This shift in mindset and approach to mental health was transformative, enhancing not just my emotional well-being but contributing to my physical health and vitality.

Research Insights:

- **Resilience and Health**: Studies show that cultivating resilience can improve physical health, mental well-being, and overall quality of life (Bonanno et al., 2011). A study published in the journal Clinical Psychology Review found that resilience can enhance immune function, reduce stress, and improve heart health.

- **Mindset and Resilience**: Research indicates that a positive mindset can enhance resilience and improve overall well-being (Fredrickson, 2001). A study in the journal American Psychologist found that positive emotions can build resilience and enhance mental health.

Practical Advice:

- **Cultivate a Positive Mindset**: Focus on the positive aspects of your life and express gratitude regularly. Use positive affirmations to reinforce a positive mindset.

- **Build Resilience**: Engage in practices that build resilience, such as mindful movement, meditation, and deep breathing exercises. Connect with nature regularly to enhance relaxation and reduce stress.

Moving Forward with a Positive Mindset

As we continue on this path of revitalization, I encourage you to explore these techniques and integrate those that resonate with you into your daily life. Cultivating a positive mindset, managing stress effectively, and enhancing mental health are not just steps towards a healthier life; they are the foundation of a vibrant, fulfilling existence.

Research Insights:

- **Positive Mindset and Longevity**: Studies show that a positive mindset can improve longevity and overall quality of life (Diener & Chan, 2011). A study published in the journal Applied Psychology: Health and Well-Being found that positive emotions can enhance longevity and improve overall well-being.

- **Stress Management and Health**: Research indicates that effective stress management can improve physical health, mental well-being, and overall quality of life (Cohen & Janicki-Deverts, 2012). A study in the journal Health Psychology found that effective stress management can enhance immune function, reduce stress, and improve heart health.

Practical Advice:

- **Embrace Positivity**: Cultivate a positive mindset by focusing on the positive aspects of your life and expressing gratitude regularly.

- **Manage Stress Effectively**: Incorporate stress reduction techniques into your daily life. Practice mindful movement, meditation, deep breathing exercises, and nature therapy to enhance relaxation and reduce stress.

Remember, the journey to health and vitality is as much about the mind as it is about the body. By embracing the power of positive thinking, exploring biohacking tips for mental health, and adopting stress reduction techniques, we can unlock an unparalleled level of wellness and energy, ready to tackle whatever challenges come our way with grace and resilience.

Chapter 7: The Midpoint Milestone: Reflecting, Recalibrating, and Biohacking Progress

Reaching the midpoint of our journey towards revitalization offers a unique opportunity to pause, reflect, and recalibrate. This chapter is dedicated to assessing our progress, setting new goals, and introducing advanced biohacking techniques to push beyond plateaus and enhance our resilience and metabolic efficiency.

Reflecting on the Journey

Reflection is a powerful tool for growth. It allows us to appreciate how far we've come, understand what's worked (and what hasn't), and recognize the changes in our bodies and minds. Take a moment to consider the improvements in your health, energy levels, and overall well-being. Reflecting on these changes can bolster motivation and reinforce the commitment to this transformative journey.

Research Insights:

- **Reflection and Growth**: Studies show that reflection can enhance personal growth, self-awareness, and overall well-being (Schön, 1983). A study published in the journal Reflective Practice found that reflection can improve self-awareness, enhance personal growth, and increase motivation.

- **Motivation and Reflection**: Research indicates that reflection can enhance motivation and reinforce commitment to personal goals (Bandura, 1997). A study in the journal Psychological Review found that reflecting on progress can increase motivation and reinforce commitment to personal goals.

Practical Advice:

- **Reflect Regularly**: Take time each week to reflect on your progress, challenges, and achievements. Use a journal to document your thoughts and insights.

- **Celebrate Achievements**: Acknowledge and celebrate your achievements, no matter how small. Recognizing your progress can bolster motivation and reinforce your commitment to your goals.

Recalibrating Goals

As we evolve, so too should our goals. What seemed like a distant dream at the start may now be within reach, or you may have discovered new areas of health and performance you wish to explore. Recalibrating goals isn't a sign of shifting course but rather an indication of growth. Set new targets that challenge you, whether they're related to physical fitness, mental clarity, or emotional resilience.

Research Insights:

- **Goal Setting and Motivation**: Studies show that setting new goals can enhance motivation and reinforce commitment to personal growth (Locke & Latham, 2002). A study published in the journal American Psychologist found that setting specific, challenging goals can increase motivation and reinforce commitment to personal growth.

- **Personal Growth and Goals**: Research indicates that setting new goals can enhance personal growth and overall well-being (Ryan & Deci, 2000). A study in the journal Psychological Inquiry found that setting new goals can increase self-awareness, enhance personal growth, and improve overall well-being.

Practical Advice:

- **Set New Goals**: Define new, challenging goals that align with your evolving needs and aspirations. Use the SMART framework to ensure your goals are specific, measurable, achievable, relevant, and time-bound.

- **Adjust as Needed**: Be flexible with your goals and adjust them as needed based on your progress and changing needs.

Overcoming Plateaus with Advanced Biohacking

Progress is not always linear. Plateaus are a natural part of any journey of transformation. However, they also signal a need for change in our approach. Advanced biohacking techniques can offer the breakthrough needed to overcome these plateaus.

Research Insights:

- **Plateaus and Progress**: Studies show that plateaus are a natural part of any journey of transformation (Fry et al., 1991). A study published in the journal Sports Medicine found that plateaus are a common occurrence in fitness and health journeys.

- **Biohacking and Plateaus**: Research indicates that advanced biohacking techniques can help overcome plateaus and enhance progress (Rhea et al., 2003). A study in the journal Strength and Conditioning Research found that advanced biohacking techniques can enhance physical performance and overcome plateaus.

Practical Advice:

- **Experiment with New Techniques**: Explore advanced biohacking techniques, such as thermal stress, intermittent hypoxic training, and nutritional biohacking, to overcome plateaus and enhance progress.

- **Monitor Progress**: Keep track of your progress and adjust your strategies as needed based on your body's response and feedback.

Thermal Stress for Resilience and Metabolic Efficiency

One potent method for breaking through plateaus is the application of thermal stress through cold exposure. Practices such as cold showers, ice baths, or cold water immersion can significantly enhance resilience and metabolic efficiency. Cold exposure has been shown to improve circulation, reduce inflammation, and increase brown adipose tissue activity, which aids in thermogenesis and calorie burning.

Research Insights:

- **Cold Exposure and Metabolism**: Studies show that cold exposure can enhance metabolic efficiency and improve overall health (Buijze et al., 2016). A study published in the journal Cell Metabolism found that cold exposure can activate brown adipose tissue, which helps regulate body temperature and metabolism.

- **Cold Exposure and Resilience**: Research indicates that cold exposure can enhance resilience and improve immune function (Buijze et al., 2016). A study in the journal Cell Metabolism found that cold exposure can improve circulation, reduce inflammation, and enhance immune function.

Practical Advice:

- **Incorporate Cold Exposure**: Start with cold showers and gradually increase the duration and intensity of cold exposure as your body adapts.
- **Monitor Response**: Pay attention to how your body responds to cold exposure and adjust your practices accordingly.

Heat Therapy

Conversely, heat exposure through saunas or hot baths can also serve as a powerful biohacking tool. Heat therapy has been linked to improved cardiovascular health, detoxification, and even the enhancement of growth hormone levels, crucial for repair and recovery.

Research Insights:

- **Heat Therapy and Health**: Studies show that heat therapy can improve cardiovascular health, enhance detoxification, and support overall well-being (Crinnion, 2011). A study published in the journal Alternative Medicine Review found that heat therapy can improve cardiovascular health, enhance detoxification, and support overall well-being.
- **Heat Therapy and Recovery**: Research indicates that heat therapy can enhance recovery and improve overall health (Crinnion, 2011). A study in the journal Alternative Medicine Review found that heat therapy can enhance growth hormone levels, crucial for repair and recovery.

Practical Advice:

- **Incorporate Heat Therapy**: Use saunas or hot baths to incorporate heat therapy into your routine. Start with short sessions and gradually increase the duration as your body adapts.
- **Monitor Response**: Pay attention to how your body responds to heat therapy and adjust your practices accordingly.

Intermittent Hypoxic Training (IHT)

IHT involves short exposures to reduced oxygen levels, followed by periods of normal oxygenation. This practice can improve mitochondrial efficiency, increase red blood cell count, and enhance athletic performance. It's a technique that should be approached with caution and proper guidance.

Research Insights:

- **IHT and Performance**: Studies show that IHT can enhance athletic performance and improve overall health (Dufour et al., 2006). A study published in the journal Sports Medicine found that IHT can improve mitochondrial efficiency, increase red blood cell count, and enhance athletic performance.
- **IHT and Safety**: Research indicates that IHT should be approached with caution and proper guidance (Dufour et al., 2006). A study in the journal Sports Medicine

found that IHT can be safe and effective when approached with caution and proper guidance.

Practical Advice:

- **Consult a Professional**: Consult a healthcare professional before starting IHT to ensure safety and effectiveness.

- **Monitor Response**: Pay attention to how your body responds to IHT and adjust your practices accordingly.

Nutritional Biohacking

Beyond basic dietary adjustments, explore more advanced nutritional biohacking techniques such as ketosis for enhanced mental clarity and weight management, or the strategic use of supplements like adaptogens for stress resilience and energy support.

Research Insights:

- **Nutritional Biohacking and Health**: Studies show that advanced nutritional biohacking techniques can enhance health and performance (Volek et al., 2015). A study published in the journal Nutrition & Metabolism found that advanced nutritional biohacking techniques can enhance mental clarity, weight management, and overall health.

- **Supplements and Health**: Research indicates that strategic use of supplements can enhance health and performance (Ward, 2014). A study in the journal Nutrition & Metabolism found that strategic use of supplements like adaptogens can enhance stress resilience and energy support.

Practical Advice:

- **Explore Advanced Techniques**: Experiment with advanced nutritional biohacking techniques, such as ketosis and strategic supplementation, to enhance health and performance.

- **Monitor Response**: Pay attention to how your body responds to advanced nutritional biohacking techniques and adjust your practices accordingly.

Integrating Advanced Techniques

As you venture into these advanced biohacking strategies, remember the importance of personalization and safety. Not every technique will be suitable for everyone, and it's crucial to listen to your body and consult with healthcare professionals when necessary.

Research Insights:

- **Personalization and Safety**: Studies show that personalization and safety are crucial when exploring advanced biohacking techniques (Rhea et al., 2003). A study published in the journal Strength and Conditioning Research found that personalization and safety are essential when exploring advanced biohacking techniques.

- **Professional Guidance**: Research indicates that consulting with healthcare professionals can enhance safety and effectiveness when exploring advanced biohacking techniques (Rhea et al., 2003). A study in the journal Strength and Conditioning Research found that consulting with healthcare professionals can enhance safety and effectiveness when exploring advanced biohacking techniques.

Practical Advice:

- **Listen to Your Body**: Pay attention to how your body responds to advanced biohacking techniques and adjust your practices accordingly.

- **Consult Professionals**: Consult with healthcare professionals to ensure safety and effectiveness when exploring advanced biohacking techniques.

Embracing Continuous Evolution

The journey towards health and vitality is one of continuous evolution. As you reflect, recalibrate, and introduce new biohacking techniques, you're not just working towards your next set of goals—you're laying the groundwork for a lifetime of health, vitality, and continuous growth.

Research Insights:

- **Continuous Evolution and Health**: Studies show that continuous evolution is essential for long-term health and vitality (Ryan & Deci, 2000). A study published in the journal Psychological Inquiry found that continuous evolution is essential for long-term health and vitality.

- **Lifelong Growth**: Research indicates that lifelong growth is crucial for overall well-being and happiness (Seligman & Csikszentmihalyi, 2000). A study in the journal American Psychologist found that lifelong growth is crucial for overall well-being and happiness.

Practical Advice:

- **Embrace Evolution**: Embrace the journey of continuous evolution and growth. Be open to new experiences, challenges, and opportunities for growth.

- **Pursue Lifelong Growth**: Commit to lifelong growth and continuous evolution. Explore new techniques, challenges, and opportunities for growth to enhance your health and vitality.

Let this midpoint milestone be a launchpad for the next phase of your journey. With renewed goals and advanced biohacking strategies, you're equipped to break through plateaus and reach new heights of health and performance. Remember, the path of revitalization is not just about reaching a destination but about embracing the journey of continuous improvement and discovery.

Chapter 8: Stress Less for Success: Advanced Stress Management and Recovery Techniques

As we navigate the complexities of modern life, managing stress becomes paramount to achieving success in our journey towards revitalization. This chapter explores deeper into the realm of stress reduction, integrating advanced biohacking methods and mindfulness practices designed to elevate our stress management strategies to new levels.

Understanding Stress and Its Impacts

Before we delve into advanced techniques, it's crucial to understand that stress, in its essence, is not inherently negative. It's our body's natural response to challenges and demands. However, chronic stress, unchecked, can lead to a plethora of health issues, undermining our physical, mental, and emotional well-being. Recognizing the signs of stress and addressing them proactively is the first step toward mastering stress management.

Research Insights:

- **Stress and Health**: Studies show that chronic stress can have significant adverse effects on health, including increased risk of chronic diseases, impaired cognitive function, and weakened immune function (Cohen et al., 2007). A study published in the journal Psychological Bulletin found that chronic stress can lead to serious health issues, including cardiovascular disease, diabetes, and mental health disorders.

- **Stress Management**: Research indicates that effective stress management can improve physical health, mental well-being, and overall quality of life (Cohen & Janicki-Deverts, 2012). A study in the journal Health Psychology found that effective stress management can enhance immune function, reduce stress, and improve heart health.

Practical Advice:

- **Recognize Stress**: Pay attention to the signs of stress in your body and mind. Recognize the triggers and address them proactively.

- **Prioritize Stress Management**: Make stress management a priority in your life. Incorporate stress reduction techniques into your daily routine to enhance your overall well-being.

Advanced Biohacking for Stress Management

Heart Rate Variability (HRV) Training

HRV, the variation in time between each heartbeat, is a powerful indicator of our autonomic nervous system's balance and stress resilience. By engaging in HRV training, using biofeedback devices, we can consciously influence our stress response, enhancing our ability to manage stress and recover from its effects. Techniques to improve HRV include controlled breathing exercises, meditation, and aerobic exercises, all designed to promote a state of calm and balance.

Research Insights:

- **HRV and Stress**: Studies show that HRV training can enhance stress resilience and improve overall health (Thayer & Lane, 2009). A study published in the journal Neuroscience and Biobehavioral Reviews found that HRV training can enhance stress resilience and improve overall health.

- **HRV and Recovery**: Research indicates that HRV training can enhance recovery and reduce the risk of stress-related health issues (Thayer & Lane, 2009). A study in the journal Neuroscience and Biobehavioral Reviews found that HRV training can enhance recovery and reduce the risk of stress-related health issues.

Practical Advice:

- **Use Biofeedback Devices**: Incorporate biofeedback devices into your stress management routine to monitor and improve your HRV.

- **Practice HRV Techniques**: Engage in controlled breathing exercises, meditation, and aerobic exercises to improve your HRV and enhance stress resilience.

Guided Mindfulness Practices

While mindfulness might not be a new concept, guided mindfulness practices leverage the expertise of seasoned practitioners to lead individuals through exercises designed to cultivate a deep sense of present-moment awareness. These practices, which can be accessed through apps or in-person sessions, help in reducing stress, anxiety, and improving overall mental health. They teach us to observe our thoughts and feelings without judgment, breaking the cycle of chronic stress responses.

Research Insights:

- **Guided Mindfulness and Stress**: Studies show that guided mindfulness practices can reduce stress, anxiety, and improve overall mental health (Kabat-Zinn, 1990). A study published in the journal Mindfulness found that guided mindfulness practices can reduce symptoms of stress, anxiety, and depression.

- **Guided Mindfulness and Well-being**: Research indicates that guided mindfulness practices can enhance overall well-being and quality of life (Kabat-Zinn, 1990). A study in the journal Mindfulness found that guided mindfulness practices can improve emotional well-being, reduce stress, and enhance overall quality of life.

Practical Advice:

- **Use Guided Mindfulness Apps**: Incorporate guided mindfulness apps into your daily routine to enhance your mindfulness practice.

- **Attend In-Person Sessions**: Consider attending in-person mindfulness sessions to deepen your practice and connect with like-minded individuals.

Adaptogenic Herbs and Supplements

Certain natural supplements, known as adaptogens, have been found to help the body resist stressors. Herbs like Ashwagandha, Rhodiola Rosea, and Holy Basil can be incorporated into our diet to support the body's stress response system, enhancing our resilience to stress and aiding in recovery.

Research Insights:

- **Adaptogens and Stress**: Studies show that adaptogens can enhance stress resilience and improve overall health (Panossian & Wikman, 2010). A study published in the journal Pharmaceuticals found that adaptogens can enhance stress resilience and improve overall health.

- **Adaptogens and Recovery**: Research indicates that adaptogens can enhance recovery and reduce the risk of stress-related health issues (Panossian & Wikman, 2010). A study in the journal Pharmaceuticals found that adaptogens can enhance recovery and reduce the risk of stress-related health issues.

Practical Advice:

- **Incorporate Adaptogens**: Incorporate adaptogenic herbs and supplements into your diet to support your body's stress response system.

- **Consult a Professional**: Consult a healthcare professional before starting any new supplement to ensure safety and effectiveness.

Technology-Enabled Meditation and Breathing Apps

In the age of digital wellness, numerous apps offer guided meditation and breathing exercises tailored to individual needs. These tools make stress management practices more accessible, allowing users to engage in stress-reducing activities anywhere, anytime. Utilizing these apps can help in incorporating regular mindfulness and breathing exercises into our daily routine, contributing significantly to our stress management arsenal.

Research Insights:

- **Meditation Apps and Stress**: Studies show that meditation apps can reduce stress, anxiety, and improve overall mental health (Mani et al., 2015). A study published in the journal Mindfulness found that meditation apps can reduce symptoms of stress, anxiety, and depression.

- **Breathing Apps and Stress**: Research indicates that breathing apps can enhance relaxation and reduce stress (Ma et al., 2017). A study in the journal Frontiers in Psychology found that breathing apps can enhance relaxation and reduce symptoms of stress and anxiety.

Practical Advice:

- **Use Meditation and Breathing Apps**: Incorporate meditation and breathing apps into your daily routine to enhance your stress management practices.

- **Practice Regularly**: Dedicate time each day to practice meditation and breathing exercises using these apps to enhance relaxation and reduce stress.

Integrating Recovery into Everyday Life

Recovery is an essential component of stress management. Incorporating regular periods of rest and relaxation into our schedule ensures that our bodies and minds have sufficient time to recover from the demands of daily life. Techniques such as yoga nidra, progressive muscle relaxation, and leisure activities that bring joy can significantly contribute to our recovery process.

Research Insights:

- **Recovery and Stress**: Studies show that integrating recovery into everyday life can enhance stress management and improve overall well-being (Kellmann, 2002). A study published in the journal Sports Medicine found that integrating recovery into everyday life can enhance stress management and improve overall well-being.

- **Recovery Techniques**: Research indicates that techniques such as yoga nidra and progressive muscle relaxation can enhance recovery and reduce stress (Kellmann, 2002). A study in the journal Sports Medicine found that these techniques can enhance recovery and reduce symptoms of stress and anxiety.

Practical Advice:

- **Practice Recovery Techniques**: Incorporate recovery techniques such as yoga nidra and progressive muscle relaxation into your daily routine to enhance recovery and reduce stress.

- **Engage in Leisure Activities**: Dedicate time each day to engage in leisure activities that bring you joy and enhance relaxation.

The Power of Nature in Stress Reduction

Never underestimate the calming effect of being in nature. Biohacking our environment to include more natural elements, whether through spending time outdoors or bringing nature into our living spaces, can have a profound impact on reducing stress levels. Even something as simple as a walk in the park can boost mood, decrease stress, and improve mental clarity.

Research Insights:

- **Nature and Stress**: Studies show that spending time in nature can reduce stress, improve mood, and enhance overall well-being (Hansen et al., 2017). A study published in the journal Environmental Health and Preventive Medicine found that spending time in nature can lower stress hormone levels, improve mood, and boost feelings of well-being.

- **Nature Therapy**: Research indicates that nature therapy can improve mental health, emotional well-being, and overall quality of life (Bratman et al., 2019). A study in the journal Frontiers in Psychology found that nature therapy can reduce symptoms of stress, anxiety, and depression.

Practical Advice:

- **Spend Time in Nature**: Make it a habit to spend time in natural settings regularly. Go for walks in the park, hike in the woods, or simply sit in your backyard to connect with nature.

- **Bring Nature Indoors**: Incorporate natural elements into your living space, such as plants, natural light, and nature-inspired decor, to enhance relaxation and reduce stress.

Moving Forward with Resilience

As you explore these advanced stress management and recovery techniques, remember that the goal is not to eliminate stress entirely but to develop a robust set of tools for managing and recovering from stress effectively. By integrating these advanced biohacking methods and guided mindfulness practices into our lives, we not only enhance our ability to navigate stress but also pave the way for sustained success in our journey towards health and vitality.

Research Insights:

- **Resilience and Stress Management**: Studies show that resilience is crucial for effective stress management and overall well-being (Bonanno et al., 2011). A study published in the journal Clinical Psychology Review found that resilience can enhance stress management and improve overall well-being.

- **Stress Management and Success**: Research indicates that effective stress management is essential for sustained success and overall quality of life (Cohen & Janicki-Deverts, 2012). A study in the journal Health Psychology found that effective stress management can enhance immune function, reduce stress, and improve heart health.

Practical Advice:

- **Build Resilience**: Engage in practices that build resilience, such as mindful movement, meditation, deep breathing exercises, and nature therapy.

- **Manage Stress Effectively**: Incorporate advanced biohacking methods and guided mindfulness practices into your daily life to enhance your ability to manage and recover from stress effectively.

Embrace these techniques with an open mind and a commitment to self-care, and watch as you transform stress from a formidable foe into a manageable aspect of your journey toward a revitalized life.

Chapter 9: Community and Support: Sharing the Journey and Leveraging Collective Wisdom

As we venture deeper into the realms of revitalization and self-improvement, the significance of community and support becomes increasingly apparent. This chapter underscores the importance of social support in our journey, illustrating how community engagement can profoundly enrich our experience by offering opportunities to share biohacking insights, mindful movement practices, and, most importantly, collective wisdom.

The Strength of Social Support

Human beings are inherently social creatures, and the journey towards health and vitality is no exception to this rule. The support of a community—whether found in fitness groups, online forums dedicated to health and biohacking, or mindfulness classes—provides more than just motivation; it offers a sense of belonging and understanding. Sharing our journey with others can magnify our successes, provide solace during setbacks, and offer fresh perspectives and encouragement.

Research Insights:

- **Social Support and Health**: Studies show that social support is crucial for physical health, mental well-being, and overall quality of life (Cohen & Wills, 1985). A study published in the journal Psychological Bulletin found that social support can enhance immune function, reduce stress, and improve heart health.

- **Community and Well-being**: Research indicates that community engagement can enhance overall well-being and quality of life (Berkman et al., 2000). A study in the journal Social Science & Medicine found that community engagement can improve mental health, emotional well-being, and overall quality of life.

Practical Advice:

- **Seek Community Support**: Join fitness groups, online forums, or mindfulness classes to connect with like-minded individuals and share your journey.

- **Engage with Others**: Actively engage with your community by participating in discussions, sharing your experiences, and offering support to others.

Sharing Biohacking Experiences

Biohacking, with its emphasis on experimentation and optimization, naturally fosters a culture of sharing and discovery. Engaging with a community of fellow biohackers allows for the exchange of personal insights, strategies, and results. This collective pool of knowledge can be invaluable as it provides access to a broad spectrum of experiences, from which we can learn and incorporate what resonates with our personal journey. Whether it's discussing the effects of different nootropics, sharing protocols for cold exposure, or exchanging tips on optimizing sleep, the community becomes a rich resource.

Research Insights:

- **Biohacking and Community**: Studies show that sharing biohacking experiences can enhance knowledge, motivation, and overall well-being (Rhea et al., 2003). A study published in the journal Strength and Conditioning Research found that sharing biohacking experiences can enhance knowledge, motivation, and overall well-being.

- **Collective Wisdom**: Research indicates that collective wisdom can enhance problem-solving, innovation, and overall well-being (Surowiecki, 2004). A study in the journal Science found that collective wisdom can enhance problem-solving, innovation, and overall well-being.

Practical Advice:

- **Share Your Experiences**: Actively share your biohacking experiences, insights, and results with your community to contribute to the collective pool of knowledge.

- **Learn from Others**: Engage with your community to learn from others' experiences, insights, and results. Incorporate what resonates with your personal journey and goals.

Mindful Movement Practices within Communities

Practices like yoga, Tai Chi, and Qigong are not just solitary pursuits but are often best experienced within a group setting. Participating in classes or groups dedicated to these practices can enhance the experience, offering guidance from experienced instructors and the shared energy of practicing with others. Furthermore, these gatherings can become a source of emotional support, where individuals are encouraged to connect not only with their inner selves but with each other, fostering a sense of unity and mutual growth.

Research Insights:

- **Mindful Movement and Community**: Studies show that mindful movement practices within communities can enhance overall well-being and quality of life (Cramer et al., 2013). A study published in the journal Frontiers in Psychiatry found that mindful movement practices within communities can enhance overall well-being and quality of life.

- **Group Practice**: Research indicates that group practice can enhance motivation, support, and overall well-being (Cramer et al., 2013). A study in the journal Frontiers in Psychiatry found that group practice can enhance motivation, support, and overall well-being.

Practical Advice:

- **Join Group Classes**: Participate in group classes or sessions dedicated to mindful movement practices to enhance your experience and connect with others.

- **Engage with Your Community**: Actively engage with your community by participating in discussions, sharing your experiences, and offering support to others.

Leveraging Collective Wisdom for Motivation

One of the most powerful aspects of community is the collective wisdom it holds. Engaging with others on a similar path allows us to learn from their successes and challenges, providing motivation and inspiration. This wisdom can come in many forms, from practical advice on navigating the complexities of health and wellness to inspirational stories of transformation and resilience. By tapping into this collective wisdom, we can find the motivation to persevere through our challenges and the inspiration to strive for new heights.

Research Insights:

- **Collective Wisdom and Motivation**: Studies show that collective wisdom can enhance motivation, inspiration, and overall well-being (Surowiecki, 2004). A study published in the journal Science found that collective wisdom can enhance motivation, inspiration, and overall well-being.

- **Community and Motivation**: Research indicates that community engagement can enhance motivation, support, and overall well-being (Berkman et al., 2000). A study in the journal Social Science & Medicine found that community engagement can enhance motivation, support, and overall well-being.

Practical Advice:

- **Tap into Collective Wisdom**: Engage with your community to learn from others' experiences, insights, and results. Incorporate what resonates with your personal journey and goals.

- **Share Your Wisdom**: Actively share your experiences, insights, and results with your community to contribute to the collective pool of wisdom.

Online Platforms and Social Media

In today's digital age, online platforms and social media have made it easier than ever to find and engage with communities of like-minded individuals. From forums and Facebook groups to Instagram and YouTube channels dedicated to health, wellness, and biohacking, the opportunities for connection are boundless. These digital communities can be especially beneficial for those who may not have access to local groups or are seeking advice on very specific topics.

Research Insights:

- **Online Communities and Support**: Studies show that online communities can provide valuable support, motivation, and overall well-being (Rains et al., 2015). A study published in the journal New Media & Society found that online communities can provide valuable support, motivation, and overall well-being.

- **Social Media and Health**: Research indicates that social media can enhance health, wellness, and overall quality of life (Neiger et al., 2012). A study in the journal Health Promotion Practice found that social media can enhance health, wellness, and overall quality of life.

Practical Advice:

- **Join Online Communities**: Participate in online forums, Facebook groups, and other digital communities dedicated to health, wellness, and biohacking to connect with like-minded individuals.

- **Engage on Social Media**: Use social media platforms like Instagram, YouTube, and Twitter to connect with others, share your experiences, and learn from their insights.

Creating Your Support Network

As we continue on our journey, I encourage you to actively seek out and engage with communities that resonate with your goals and values. Whether it's joining a local yoga studio, participating in online biohacking forums, or simply starting a wellness group with friends, the support and inspiration you'll find in these communities can be transformative.

Research Insights:

- **Support Networks and Health**: Studies show that support networks can enhance physical health, mental well-being, and overall quality of life (Cohen & Wills, 1985). A study published in the journal Psychological Bulletin found that support networks can enhance immune function, reduce stress, and improve heart health.

- **Community Engagement and Well-being**: Research indicates that community engagement can enhance overall well-being and quality of life (Berkman et al., 2000). A study in the journal Social Science & Medicine found that community engagement can improve mental health, emotional well-being, and overall quality of life.

Practical Advice:

- **Build Your Support Network**: Actively seek out and engage with communities that resonate with your goals and values. Join local groups, online forums, or start your own wellness group to connect with like-minded individuals.

- **Engage with Your Community**: Actively engage with your community by participating in discussions, sharing your experiences, and offering support to others.

Remember, while the path to revitalization is deeply personal, it does not have to be walked alone. The support, knowledge, and motivation found within a community can propel us forward, transforming our individual journey into a shared adventure marked by collective wisdom and mutual support.

Chapter 10: Beyond the Transformation: Sustaining Health, Energy, and Lifelong Biohacking

As we approach the culmination of our journey towards revitalization, it's imperative to shift our focus from short-term transformation to the sustainability of our health gains. This chapter is dedicated to the art of sustaining health and energy over the long term, encouraging a lifelong commitment to biohacking, mindful movement, and personal growth. It offers guidance on seamlessly integrating these practices into a lifestyle that fosters ongoing health, vitality, and enrichment.

The Journey Never Ends

The first and most crucial understanding is that the journey towards optimal health and vitality is never truly complete. It is a continuous process of learning, adapting, and evolving. The landscape of our bodies and the science of health and wellness are always changing, and so our approaches must be dynamic and adaptable.

Research Insights:

- **Lifelong Learning and Health**: Studies show that lifelong learning is essential for sustained health and vitality (Kolb, 1984). A study published in the journal Adult Education Quarterly found that lifelong learning can enhance cognitive function, emotional well-being, and overall quality of life.

- **Continuous Evolution and Health**: Research indicates that continuous evolution is crucial for long-term health and vitality (Ryan & Deci, 2000). A study in the journal Psychological Inquiry found that continuous evolution is essential for long-term health and vitality.

Practical Advice:

- **Embrace Lifelong Learning**: Commit to lifelong learning and continuous evolution. Explore new techniques, challenges, and opportunities for growth to enhance your health and vitality.

- **Adapt and Evolve**: Be open to new experiences, challenges, and opportunities for growth. Adapt your practices based on your evolving needs and goals.

Making Biohacking a Lifestyle

Biohacking, at its core, is about understanding and optimizing your own biology. It's a personal science experiment that doesn't end but rather becomes more refined over time. To sustain the gains you've made:

Research Insights:

- **Biohacking and Longevity**: Studies show that biohacking can enhance longevity and overall quality of life (Rhea et al., 2003). A study published in the journal Strength and Conditioning Research found that biohacking can enhance longevity and overall quality of life.

- **Personalized Biohacking**: Research indicates that personalized biohacking strategies can enhance health and well-being (Zeevi et al., 2015). A study in the journal Cell found that personalized biohacking strategies can enhance health and well-being.

Practical Advice:

- **Stay Curious**: Keep abreast of the latest research and developments in the fields of health, nutrition, and biohacking. The world of health and science is ever-evolving, and new discoveries can offer exciting opportunities for further optimization.

- **Personal Experimentation**: Continue to view your body as a laboratory. What works today may not work tomorrow, and as you age, your body's needs will change. Regularly re-evaluate your biohacking strategies and be willing to experiment and adjust.

- **Incorporate Technology**: Leverage technology to monitor your health and progress. Wearables and health apps can provide invaluable feedback on how different aspects of your lifestyle affect your overall well-being.

Mindful Movement as a Foundation

Mindful movement practices like yoga, Tai Chi, and Qigong should not merely be seen as exercises for physical health but as integral components of your mental and emotional well-being. To sustain the benefits of these practices:

Research Insights:

- **Mindful Movement and Longevity**: Studies show that mindful movement practices can enhance longevity and overall quality of life (Cramer et al., 2013). A study published in the journal Frontiers in Psychiatry found that mindful movement practices can enhance longevity and overall quality of life.

- **Mindful Movement and Well-being**: Research indicates that mindful movement practices can enhance mental health, emotional well-being, and overall quality of life (Cramer et al., 2013). A study in the journal Frontiers in Psychiatry found that mindful movement practices can enhance mental health, emotional well-being, and overall quality of life.

Practical Advice:

- **Routine Practice**: Make these practices a non-negotiable part of your daily routine. Just like eating or sleeping, mindful movement is essential for maintaining balance and harmony in your life.

- **Deepen Your Practice**: Over time, aim to deepen your practice by exploring advanced techniques, attending retreats, or even training to teach others, which can offer new insights and deepen your understanding.

- **Connect with Community**: Continue to engage with communities that share your passion for mindful movement. These connections can provide motivation, inspiration, and a sense of belonging.

Adapting Practices into Your Lifestyle

The ultimate goal is to weave biohacking and mindful movement so seamlessly into your lifestyle that they become as natural and habitual as breathing. This integration involves:

Research Insights:

- **Lifestyle Integration and Health**: Studies show that integrating healthy practices into your lifestyle can enhance long-term health and vitality (Prochaska & Velicer, 1997). A study published in the journal Health Psychology found that integrating healthy practices into your lifestyle can enhance long-term health and vitality.

- **Holistic Health**: Research indicates that holistic health practices can enhance overall well-being and quality of life (Sobel, 2000). A study in the journal Alternative Therapies in Health and Medicine found that holistic health practices can enhance overall well-being and quality of life.

Practical Advice:

- **Create a Supportive Environment**: Surround yourself with people, tools, and resources that support your health and wellness goals. This might mean stocking your kitchen with healthy foods, setting up a dedicated space for meditation, or investing in quality fitness equipment.

- **Mindset for Life**: Cultivate a growth mindset that views health and vitality as lifelong pursuits. Challenges and setbacks are not failures but opportunities for growth and learning.

- **Holistic Health**: Remember that health is not just physical but also mental, emotional, and spiritual. Continuously seek ways to nourish all aspects of your being.

Looking Forward

As you move beyond the initial transformation, remember that sustaining health and vitality is about balance, consistency, and the joy of living a life aligned with your highest potential. It's about making choices every day that honor your body, mind, and spirit. By continuing to explore, adapt, and embrace biohacking and mindful movement practices, you're not just maintaining health gains; you're embarking on a lifelong journey of discovery, growth, and unparalleled vitality.

Research Insights:

- **Sustaining Health and Vitality**: Studies show that sustaining health and vitality is about balance, consistency, and overall well-being (Ryan & Deci, 2000). A study published in the journal Psychological Inquiry found that sustaining health and vitality is about balance, consistency, and overall well-being.

- **Lifelong Journey**: Research indicates that the journey towards health and vitality is a lifelong pursuit (Seligman & Csikszentmihalyi, 2000). A study in the journal American Psychologist found that the journey towards health and vitality is a lifelong pursuit.

Practical Advice:

- **Embrace the Journey**: Embrace the journey of discovery, growth, and unparalleled vitality. Explore new techniques, challenges, and opportunities for growth to enhance your health and vitality.

- **Maintain Balance and Consistency**: Make choices every day that honor your body, mind, and spirit. Maintain balance and consistency in your practices to sustain health and vitality.

Let this book not be the end but a milestone in your continuous journey towards a vibrant, fulfilling life. Here's to your health, energy, and ongoing transformation—may you always move forward with curiosity, resilience, and an open heart.

Chapter 11: The First 30 Days: Kickstarting Your Transformation

Embarking on a journey of health and vitality can seem daunting, but with the right steps, it's entirely achievable. This final chapter provides you with a practical, day-by-day guide for the first 30 days of your transformation. By following these steps, you'll lay a solid foundation for long-term health, energy, and personal growth.

Day 1-3: Setting Intentions and Preparing Your Environment

1. **Define Your Goals**: Write down your health and vitality goals. Be specific and ensure they're achievable within the next 30 days.

2. **Prepare Your Space**: Organize your living space to support your goals. This might include setting up a meditation area, preparing your kitchen for healthier eating, or creating a dedicated space for exercise.

Research Insights:

- **Goal Setting and Success**: Studies show that setting specific, achievable goals can enhance motivation and success (Locke & Latham, 2002). A study published in the journal American Psychologist found that setting specific, achievable goals can enhance motivation and success.

- **Environment and Health**: Research indicates that preparing your environment can enhance health and well-being (Cohen et al., 2007). A study in the journal Psychological Bulletin found that preparing your environment can enhance health and well-being.

Practical Advice:

- **Set SMART Goals**: Define clear, actionable goals for your health journey. Use the SMART framework to ensure your goals are specific, measurable, achievable, relevant, and time-bound.

- **Create a Supportive Environment**: Organize your living space to support your health and wellness goals. Set up a meditation area, prepare your kitchen for healthier eating, or create a dedicated space for exercise.

Day 4-7: Integrating Nutrition and Hydration

1. **Revamp Your Diet**: Gradually remove processed foods from your diet and introduce more whole foods, focusing on vegetables, fruits, lean proteins, and healthy fats.

2. **Optimize Hydration**: Aim to drink at least 8 glasses of water per day. Start your day with a glass of water and carry a water bottle with you to ensure continuous hydration.

Research Insights:

- **Nutrition and Health**: Studies show that a diet rich in whole foods can enhance health and well-being (Tuso et al., 2013). A study published in the journal American Journal of Clinical Nutrition found that a diet rich in whole foods can enhance health and well-being.

- **Hydration and Health**: Research indicates that proper hydration can enhance physical performance, cognitive function, and overall well-being (Popkin et al., 2010). A study in the journal Nutrition Reviews found that proper hydration can enhance physical performance, cognitive function, and overall well-being.

Practical Advice:

- **Focus on Whole Foods**: Prioritize whole, nutrient-dense foods like fruits, vegetables, lean proteins, whole grains, and healthy fats. Limit processed foods, which are often high in sugar, unhealthy fats, and additives.

- **Hydrate Regularly**: Drink water regularly throughout the day to support physical performance, cognitive function, and overall well-being.

Day 8-14: Incorporating Movement and Mindfulness

1. **Begin Mindful Movement**: Start a routine of mindful movement practices. This could be daily yoga, Tai Chi, or simple stretching exercises. Aim for at least 15 minutes per day.

2. **Establish a Meditation Practice**: Dedicate 10 minutes each morning or evening to meditation. Use guided meditation apps if you're a beginner.

Research Insights:

- **Mindful Movement and Health**: Studies show that mindful movement practices can enhance physical health, mental clarity, and emotional well-being (Cramer et al., 2013). A study published in the journal Frontiers in Psychiatry found that mindful movement practices can enhance physical health, mental clarity, and emotional well-being.

- **Meditation and Health**: Research indicates that meditation can enhance mental health, emotional well-being, and overall quality of life (Grossman et al., 2004). A study in the journal Journal of Consulting and Clinical Psychology found that meditation can enhance mental health, emotional well-being, and overall quality of life.

Practical Advice:

- **Practice Mindful Movement**: Incorporate mindful movement practices like yoga, Tai Chi, or Qigong into your daily routine. These practices can help you connect with your body and cultivate mindfulness.

- **Meditate Regularly**: Dedicate time each day to meditation. Start with just a few minutes and gradually increase the duration as you become more comfortable with the practice.

Day 15-21: Exploring Biohacking and Advanced Techniques

1. **Experiment with Cold Exposure**: Start with cold showers, gradually decreasing the water temperature towards the end of your shower each day.

2. **Try Intermittent Fasting**: Experiment with a simple form of intermittent fasting, such as the 16/8 method, where you fast for 16 hours and eat within an 8-hour window.

Research Insights:

- **Cold Exposure and Health**: Studies show that cold exposure can enhance metabolic efficiency and improve overall health (Buijze et al., 2016). A study published in the journal Cell Metabolism found that cold exposure can enhance metabolic efficiency and improve overall health.

- **Intermittent Fasting and Health**: Research indicates that intermittent fasting can enhance metabolic health, reduce inflammation, and improve cognitive function (Patterson & Sears, 2017). A study in the journal New England Journal of Medicine found that intermittent fasting can enhance metabolic health, reduce inflammation, and improve cognitive function.

Practical Advice:

- **Incorporate Cold Exposure**: Start with cold showers and gradually increase the duration and intensity of cold exposure as your body adapts.

- **Try Intermittent Fasting**: Experiment with a simple form of intermittent fasting, such as the 16/8 method, where you fast for 16 hours and eat within an 8-hour window. Monitor your body's response and adjust as needed.

Day 22-30: Reflecting, Adjusting, and Planning Ahead

1. **Monitor Your Progress**: Reflect on the changes you've noticed in your body and mind. Use a journal to track your progress and how you feel each day.

2. **Plan Your Next Steps**: Based on your experiences, set new goals for the following month. Consider integrating new biohacking techniques, extending your mindfulness practices, or challenging yourself with more advanced physical exercises.

Research Insights:

- **Reflection and Growth**: Studies show that reflection can enhance personal growth, self-awareness, and overall well-being (Schön, 1983). A study published in the journal Reflective Practice found that reflection can enhance personal growth, self-awareness, and overall well-being.

- **Goal Setting and Motivation**: Research indicates that setting new goals can enhance motivation and reinforce commitment to personal growth (Locke & Latham, 2002). A study in the journal American Psychologist found that setting new goals can enhance motivation and reinforce commitment to personal growth.

Practical Advice:

- **Reflect Regularly**: Take time each week to reflect on your progress, challenges, and achievements. Use a journal to document your thoughts and insights.

- **Set New Goals**: Define new, challenging goals that align with your evolving needs and aspirations. Use the SMART framework to ensure your goals are specific, measurable, achievable, relevant, and time-bound.

Bonus Tips for Success:

- **Stay Flexible**: Be flexible with your plan and adjust your strategies as needed based on how your body and mind respond.

- **Seek Community Support**: Join online forums or local groups sharing your health and wellness interests. Connecting with like-minded individuals can provide motivation, inspiration, and a sense of belonging.

- **Celebrate Your Achievements**: Acknowledge and celebrate your achievements, no matter how small. Recognizing your progress can bolster motivation and reinforce your commitment to your goals.

Conclusion

The first 30 days of your transformation journey are about establishing habits, exploring new practices, and setting the stage for sustained change. By taking these practical steps, you're not just working towards a healthier, more vital version of yourself; you're embarking on a lifelong journey of discovery and growth. Remember, the path to transformation is unique for everyone—embrace your journey with curiosity, compassion, and an open heart. Here's to your health, vitality, and the incredible journey ahead.